First Published by Evans Brothers Limited
2A Portman Mansions,Chiltern Street, London W1U 6NR,
United Kingdom

This edition published under license from Evans Brothers
Limited

North America edition published by Chelsea Clubhouse,
a division of Chelsea House Publishers and a subsidiary of
Haights Cross Communications
2080 Cabot Boulevard West, Suite 201, Langhorne,
PA 19047-1813

Printed in China

Library of Congress Cataloging-in-Publication Data
applied for.

ISBN 0-7910-8183-4

Acknowledgments

The author and publishers would like to thank the following
for their help with this book:

Nicky, Terry, and Luke Parker, Paul Thomas and Jenny Roe,
and Space Adventure, Swindon.

Thanks also to the UK Down's Syndrome Association for
their help in the preparation of this book.

All photographs by Gareth Boden

Credits

Series Editor: Louise John
Editor: Julia Bird
Designer: Mark Holt
Production: Jenny Mulvanny

LIKE ME LIKE YOU

Luke Has
DOWN'S
SYNDROME

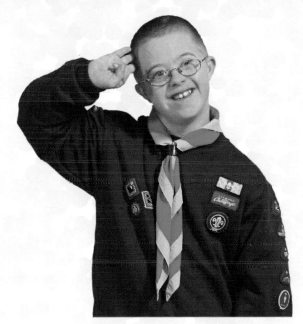

JILLIAN POWELL

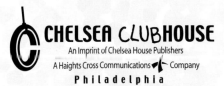

CHELSEA CLUBHOUSE
An Imprint of Chelsea House Publishers
A Haights Cross Communications Company
Philadelphia

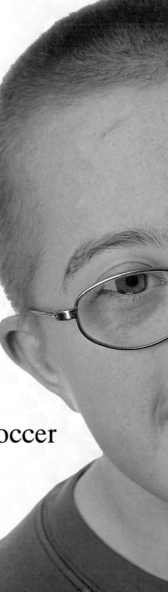

Hi, my name is Luke.
I live in England
with my Mom
and Dad and my
brothers, Kenny
and Zac. We've
got a dog called
Dana, six goldfish,
and three guinea
pigs! I like playing soccer
and tennis and going
to the movies.

I was born with **Down's syndrome**. It means I look a little different from most people and I have some **learning difficulties**.

DOWN'S SYNDROME

About one in a thousand babies is born with Down's syndrome.

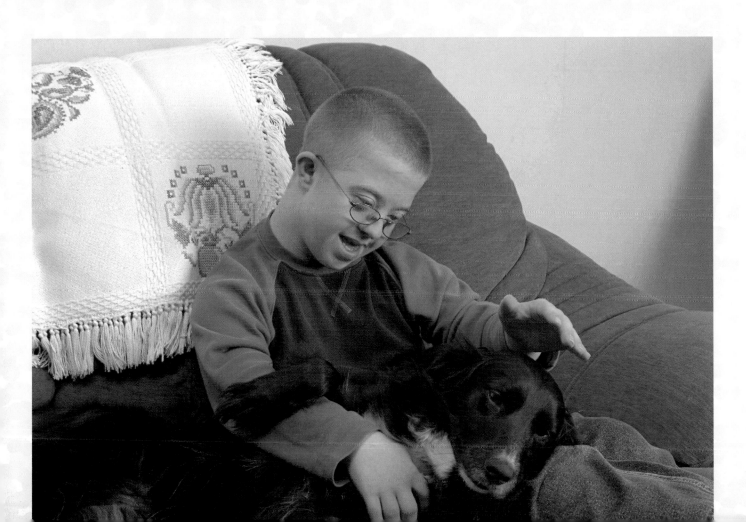

Having Down's syndrome means I sometimes need extra help with things. I like to help too, though. Today I set the table for breakfast, then I help Mom eat up the sausages!

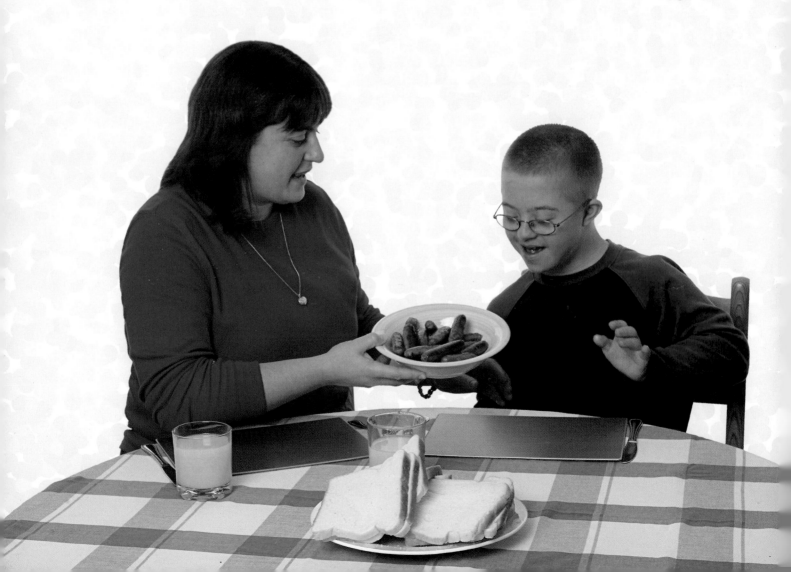

I need extra help learning words. Mom helps me at home and I have special lessons to help me talk and read at school, too. I have to pick a letter on the cards that matches the picture Mom shows me.

EXTRA HELP

Children with Down's syndrome need extra help learning to talk and read.

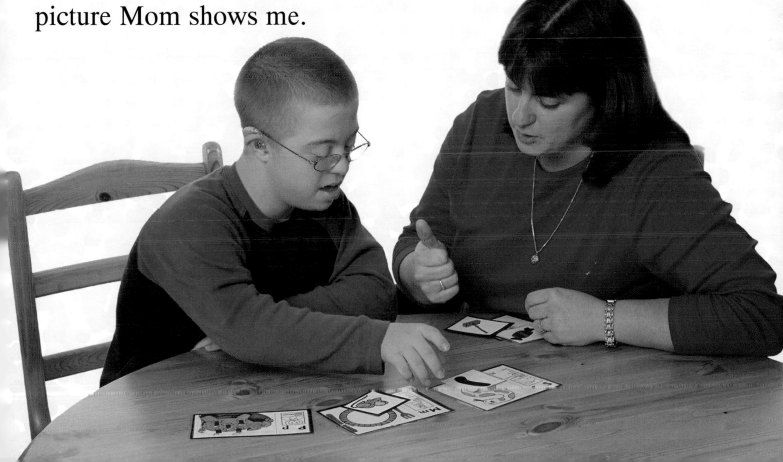

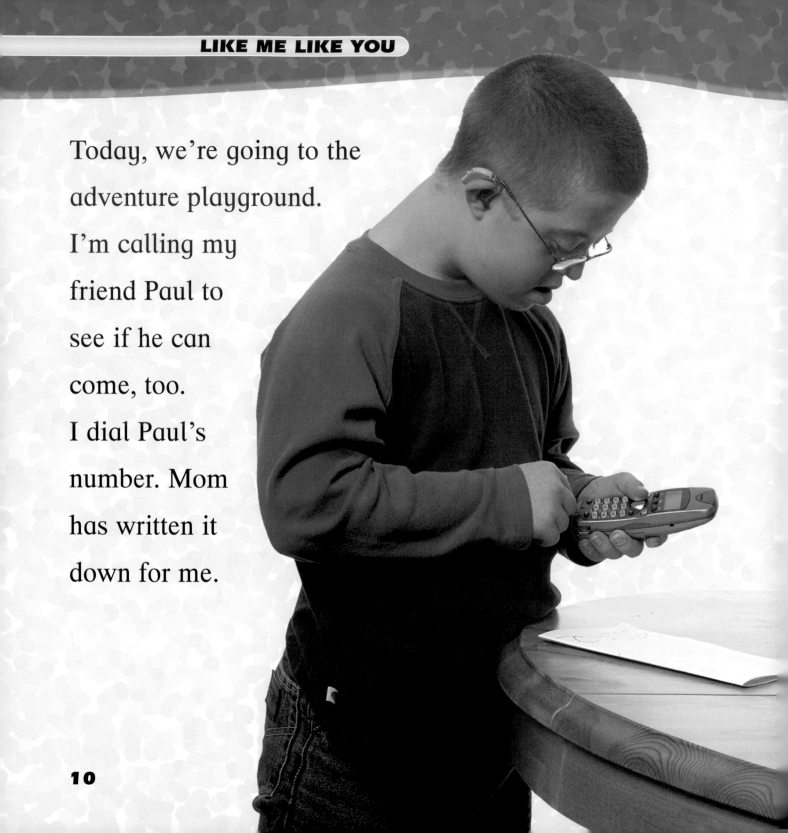

Today, we're going to the adventure playground. I'm calling my friend Paul to see if he can come, too. I dial Paul's number. Mom has written it down for me.

10

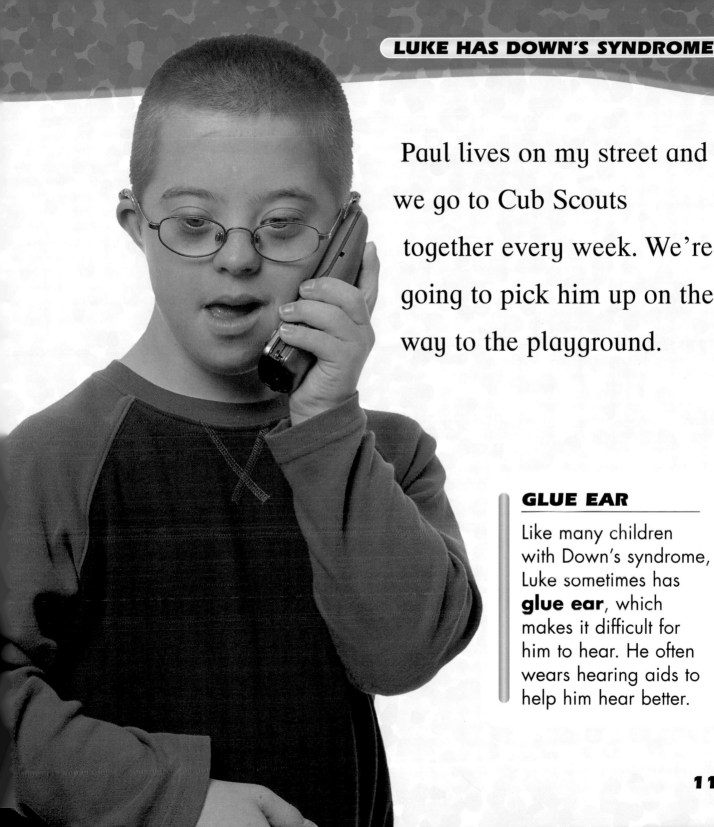

Paul lives on my street and we go to Cub Scouts together every week. We're going to pick him up on the way to the playground.

GLUE EAR

Like many children with Down's syndrome, Luke sometimes has **glue ear**, which makes it difficult for him to hear. He often wears hearing aids to help him hear better.

Mom and I walk to Paul's house to meet him. When I go out, I need help to look out for traffic and to cross the road safely.

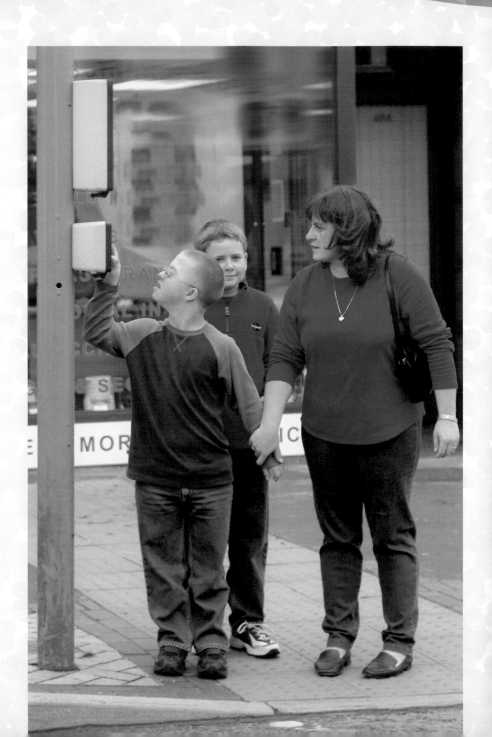

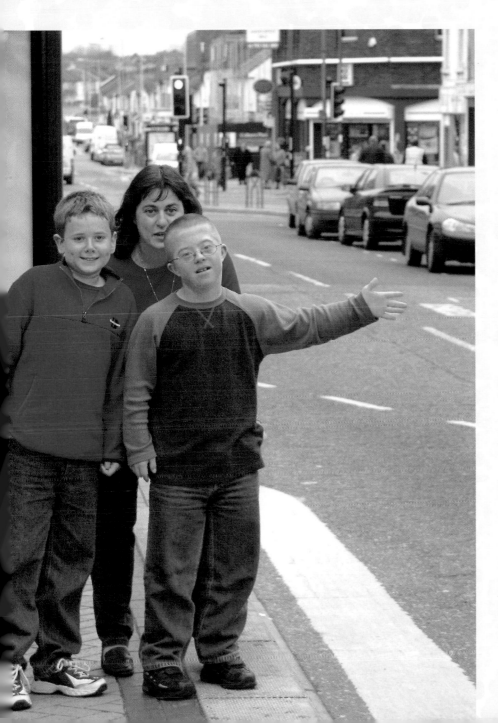

We are waiting for the bus to the adventure playground. Someone has to tell me when to put out my hand to stop the right bus!

There are lots of things to do at the adventure playground. Paul and I love going on the giant slides!

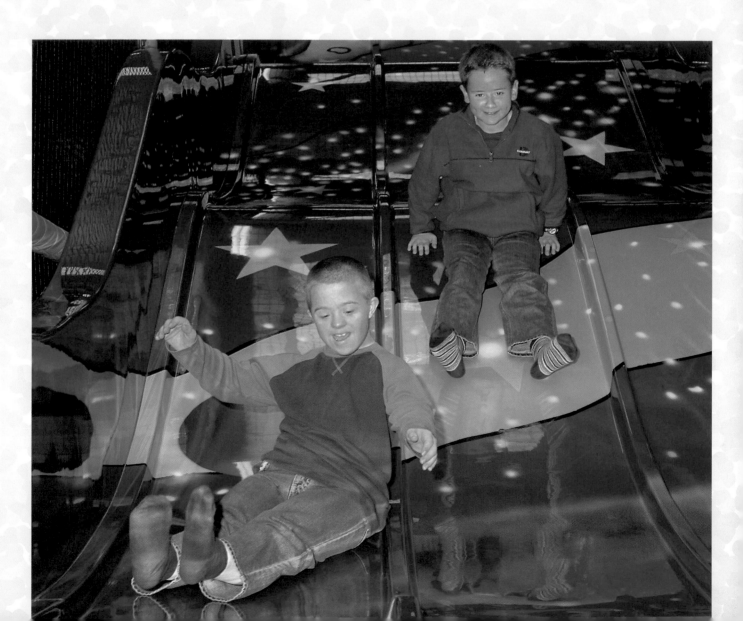

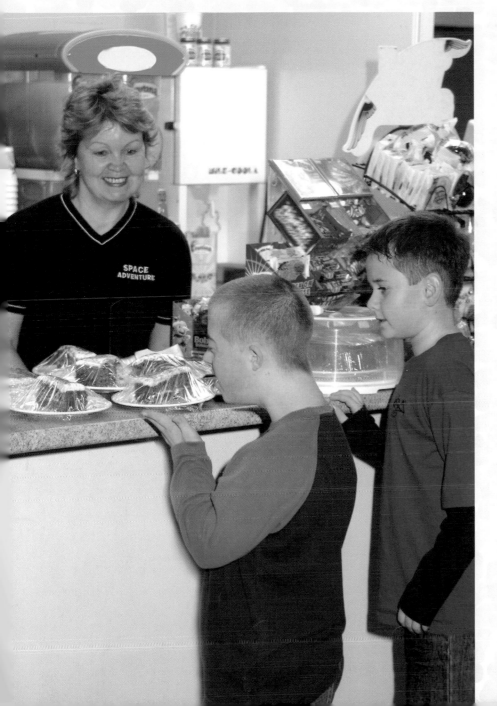

It's time for a break. We buy a drink and a snack at the restaurant. Paul helps me count out the money to pay.

Now we're trying
out the ball pool!
Paul and I practice
throwing and
catching the balls
between us.

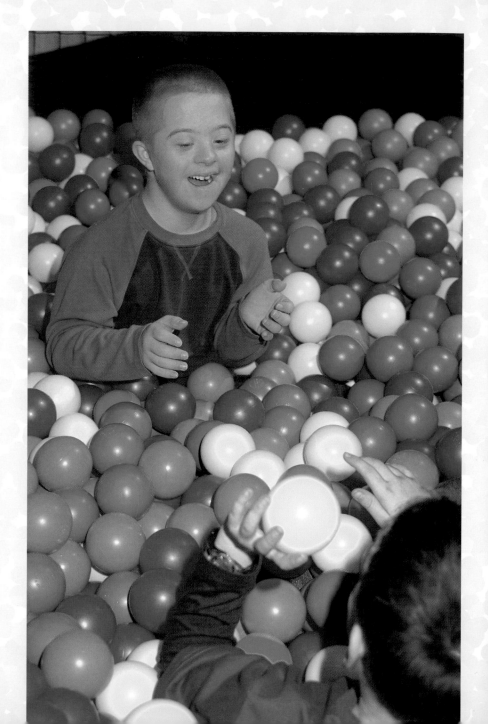

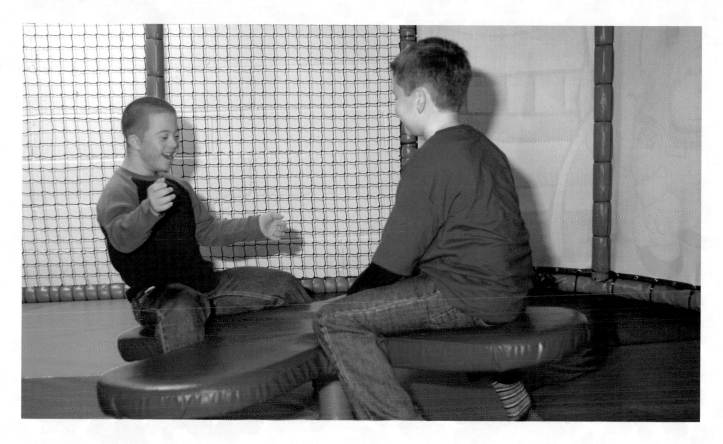

This is a kind of seesaw.
We try bouncing up and
down on it. It's lots of fun,
but I keep falling off!

Every child with Down's syndrome
is different. Some have more
learning difficulties than others.
Others have health problems with
their ears, chest, or heart.

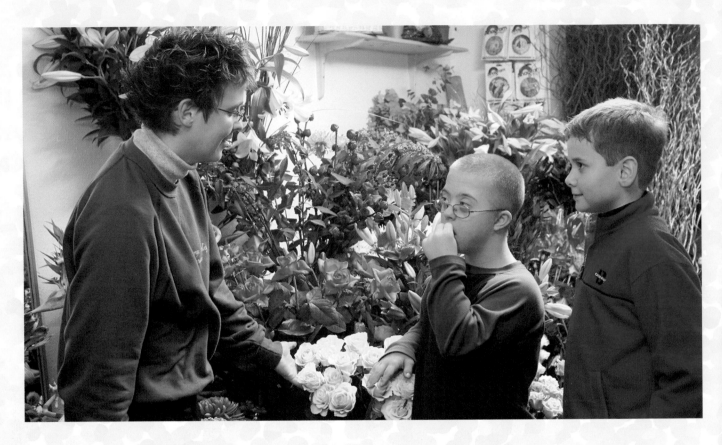

On the way home, Paul tells me it's his mom's birthday. We stop at the flower shop so we can buy her some flowers. I use **Makaton signing** to help me explain which flowers I want.

I like red flowers best, so I sign the color red. The lady helps us choose a nice bunch of flowers.

MAKATON SIGNING

Some children with Down's syndrome learn Makaton signing before they can talk. They use it to help others understand them.

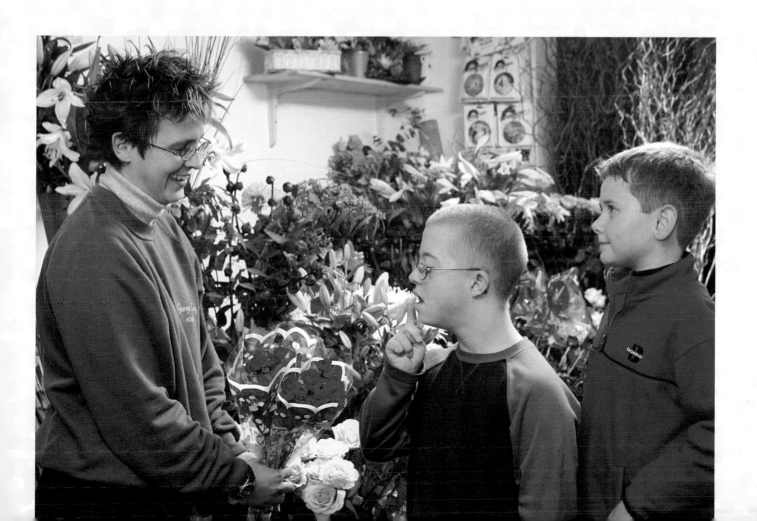

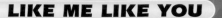

Paul and I go to Cub Scouts in the church hall once a week. I get dressed in my scout uniform. Sometimes I need a bit of help getting dressed. Dad helps me tie my scarf.

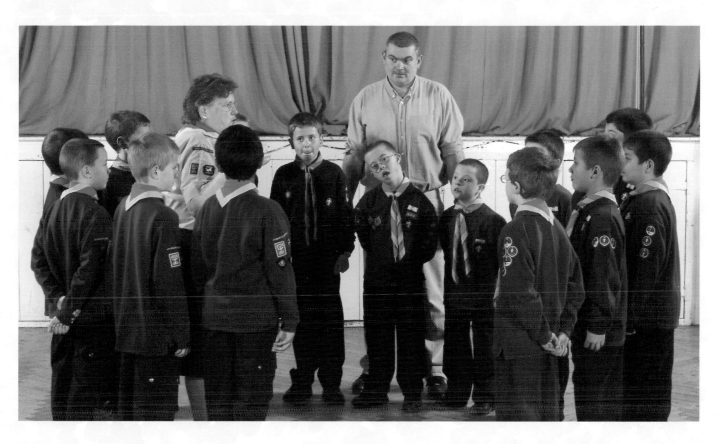

Every week, we start by raising the flag. Then the scout leader tells us what we're going to do today. Dad stands behind me to help. He says everything again, and speaks slowly and clearly so I can understand what I need to do.

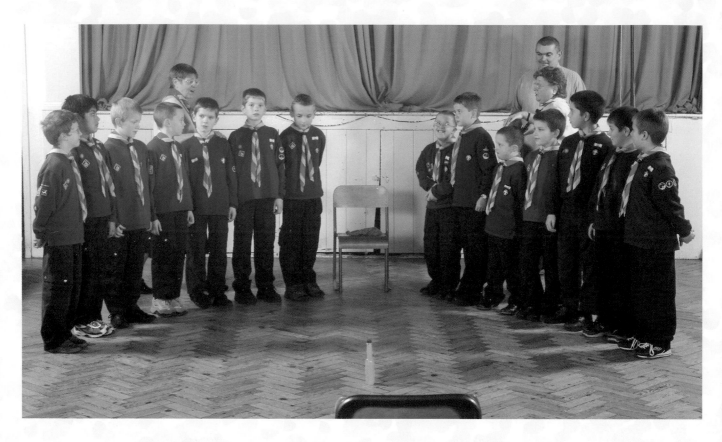

Today we're playing one of my favorite games. It's called the ball and bottle game. We get into two teams. We're each given a number, and when your number is called out you have to run to the chair.

You have to try to knock the bottle over before the scout from the other team does. The first one to knock the bottle over wins a point for his team.

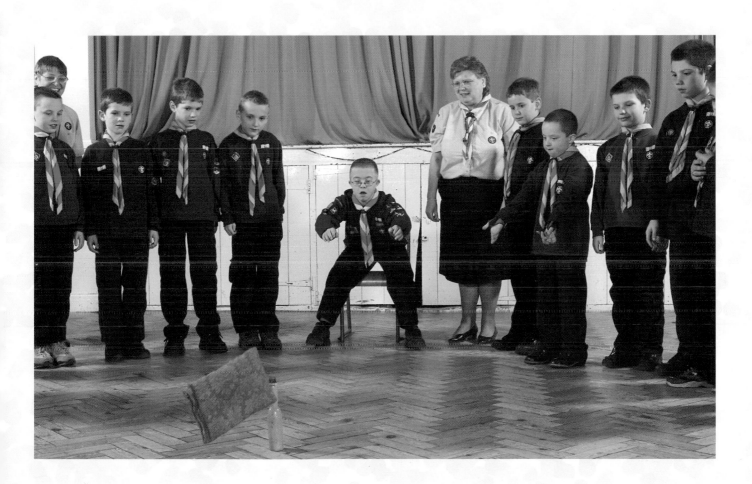

We do crafts, too. Today we've made puppets from *The Jungle Book*. I watch the other scouts to help me understand what to do. We put on a play with the puppets for the other scouts.

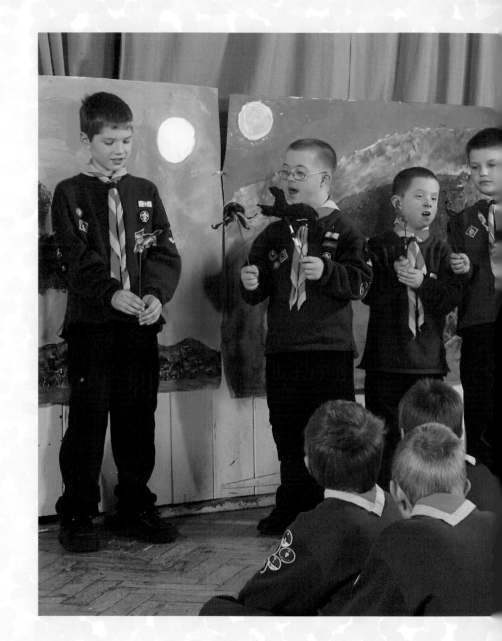

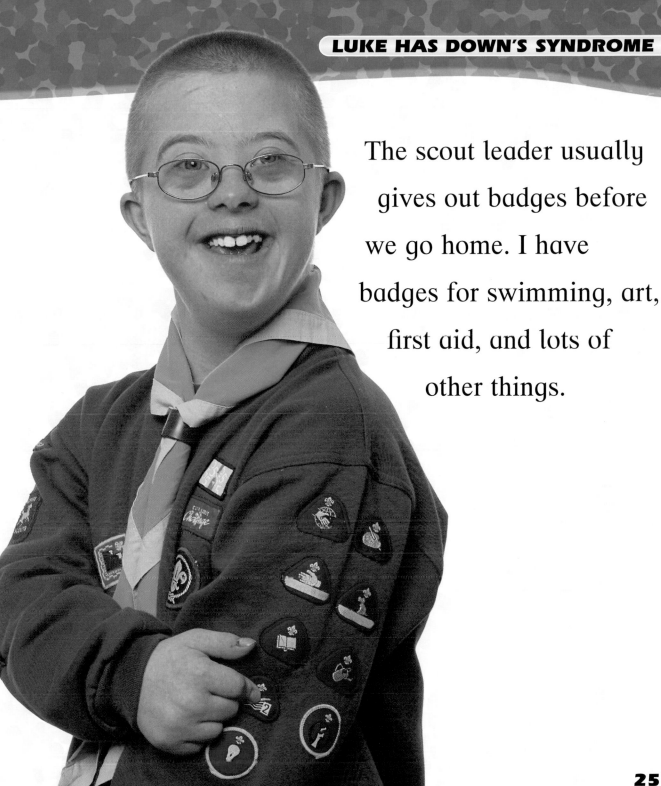

The scout leader usually gives out badges before we go home. I have badges for swimming, art, first aid, and lots of other things.

When I get home, I watch television with my brother Zac. Dad usually reads to me before I go to sleep. I can only read a few words myself but I like listening to stories, especially adventure stories.

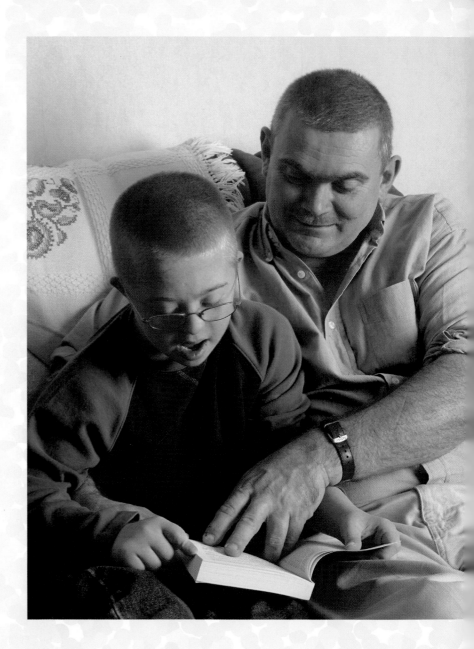

Having Down's syndrome means I need extra help with some things at home and at school. But there are lots of things I can do that I enjoy, like soccer and Cub Scouts, and taking my dog Dana for walks!

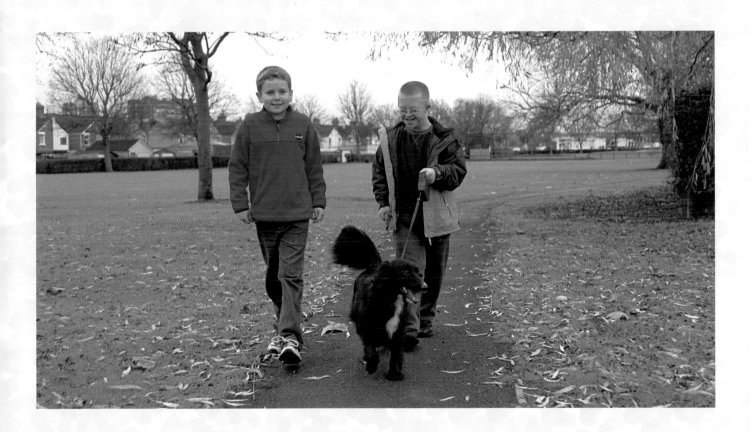

Glossary

Down's syndrome babies born with Down's syndrome have a slightly different cell makeup from most people; it affects the way they look and also gives them some learning difficulties

Glue ear a condition in which sticky fluid builds up in the ear; it can cause hearing loss, particularly in children

Learning difficulties when someone needs extra help to learn reading and writing and other skills

Makaton signing a way of making signs with the hands and face to help someone understand what you are saying

Index

Further Information

National Association for Down Syndrome (NADS)
630-325-9112
www.nads.org
Information, facts, and family stories, plus counseling and support for parents of newly diagnosed infants with Down syndrome.

Down Syndrome: For New Parents
www.downsyn.com
A resource for parents of children with Down syndrome. The site was created by a couple after their son was born with Down syndrome.

Association for Children with Down Syndrome (ACDS)
516-933-4700 ext 100
www.acds.org
Dedicated to the education and training of children with Down syndrome.

The Down Syndrome WWW Page
www.nas.com/downsyn/
This site is composed of contributions from professionals and parents who are subscribers to the Down syndrome listserv and newsgroup.

BOOKS
Focus on Down's Syndrome Research, Jeffrey A. Malard, Nova Science Publishers, Incorporated, 2004

The Five Goodbyes: Mothering My Child with Down Syndrome, Pat Ferguson Hanson, Xlibris Corporation, 2004

Yoga for Special Child Braz: A Therapeutic Approach for Infants and Children with Down Syndrome, Cerebral Palsy, Learning Disabilities, Sonia Sumar, Special Yoga Publications, 2004

The Down Syndrome Nutrition Handbook, Joan E. Guthrie Medlen, R.D., L.D., Woodbine House, 2002

A Parent's Guide to Down Syndrome, Siegfried M. Pueschel, Paul H. Brookes Publishing Company, 2001

Everything You Need to Know About Down Syndrome, Mary Bowman-Kruhm, Ed.D., Rosen Publishing Group Inc., 2000

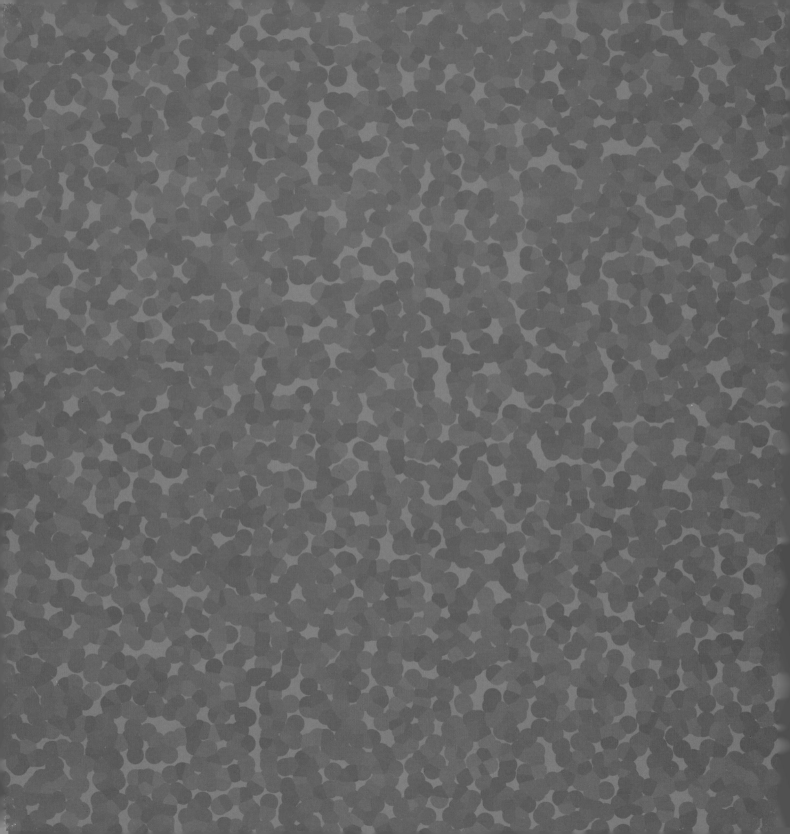